SKILLED AND VOCATIONAL TRADES

BECOME A CLINICAL LABORATORY TECHNICIAN

by Mike Downs

BrightPoint Press

San Diego, CA

BrightPoint Press

an imprint of ReferencePoint Press, Inc.
Printed in the United States

For more information, contact:
BrightPoint Press
PO Box 27779
San Diego, CA 92198
www.BrightPointPress.com

LIBRARY OF CONGRESS CATALOGING-IN-PUBLICATION DATA

Name: Downs, Mike, author.
Title: Become a clinical laboratory technician / by Mike Downs.
Description: San Diego, CA: ReferencePoint Press, 2027 | Series: Skilled and vocational trades | Includes bibliographical references and index. | Audience: Grades 7–9
Identifiers: ISBN 9781678214586 (hardcover) | ISBN 9781678214593 (eBook)
The complete Library of Congress record is available at www.loc.gov.

CONTENTS

AT A GLANCE

- Clinical lab technicians (CLTs) perform tests on bodily fluids and tissues to help identify and treat diseases.
- CLTs must learn how to use many types of tools and machines to perform tests.
- To become CLTs, people must graduate high school. They can then enroll in 2-year or 4-year programs to learn to be CLTs.
- Some CLTs specialize in specific areas. These areas can include microbiology, clinical chemistry, and hematology.
- A CLT can have a variety of schedules. Some CLTs work regular daytime hours, while others work night shifts.

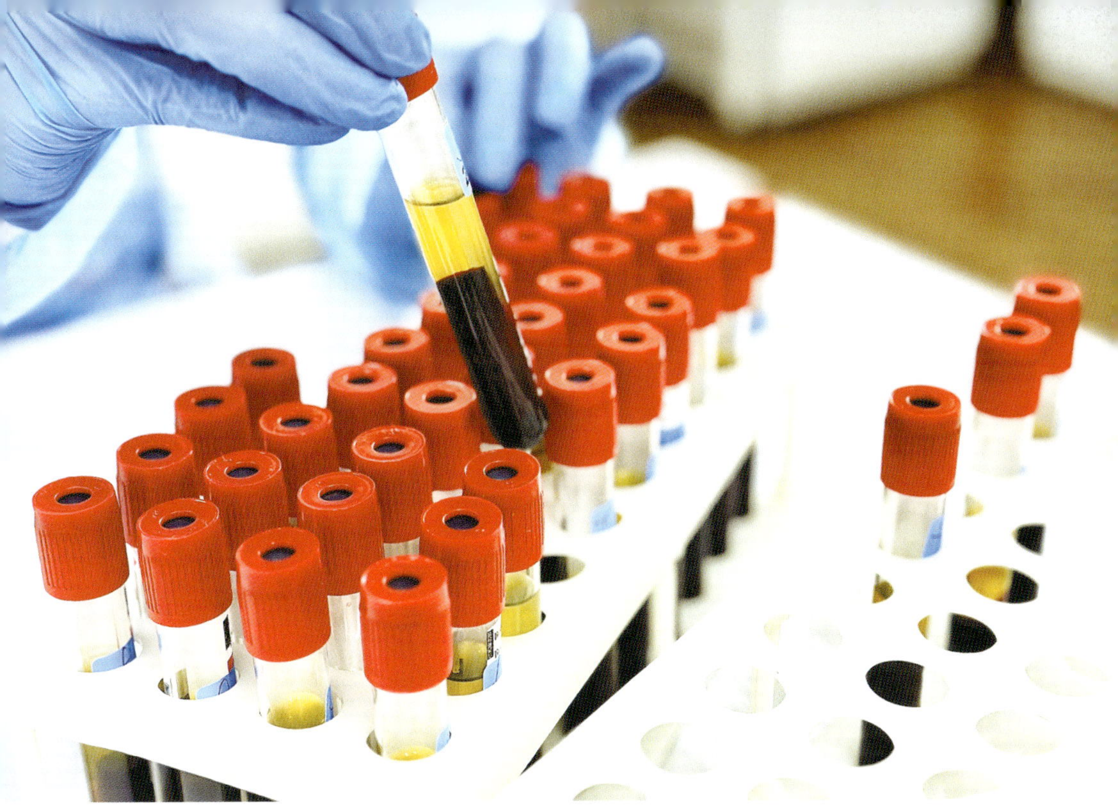

- CLTs must be comfortable working with bodily fluids. They must also be okay with seeing strange microorganisms and body parts.

- The average salary for a CLT is below the national average. But people can earn more by becoming supervisors.

- As technology changes, so will the jobs CLTs perform. However, the career's future is strong.

MEDICAL DETECTIVES

Kim Conner pushes open the door to the lab. She is greeted by clinking glass tubes and the whir of machines. This is where she works in the hospital. She is a clinical laboratory technician (CLT).

"When I come in," she says, "I check what's going on from the previous shift."[1] She needs to know if the testing machines are working. She finds all the chemicals she needs to run tests. Then her day gets busy.

Clinical laboratory technicians help hospitals provide quick and effective care for patients.

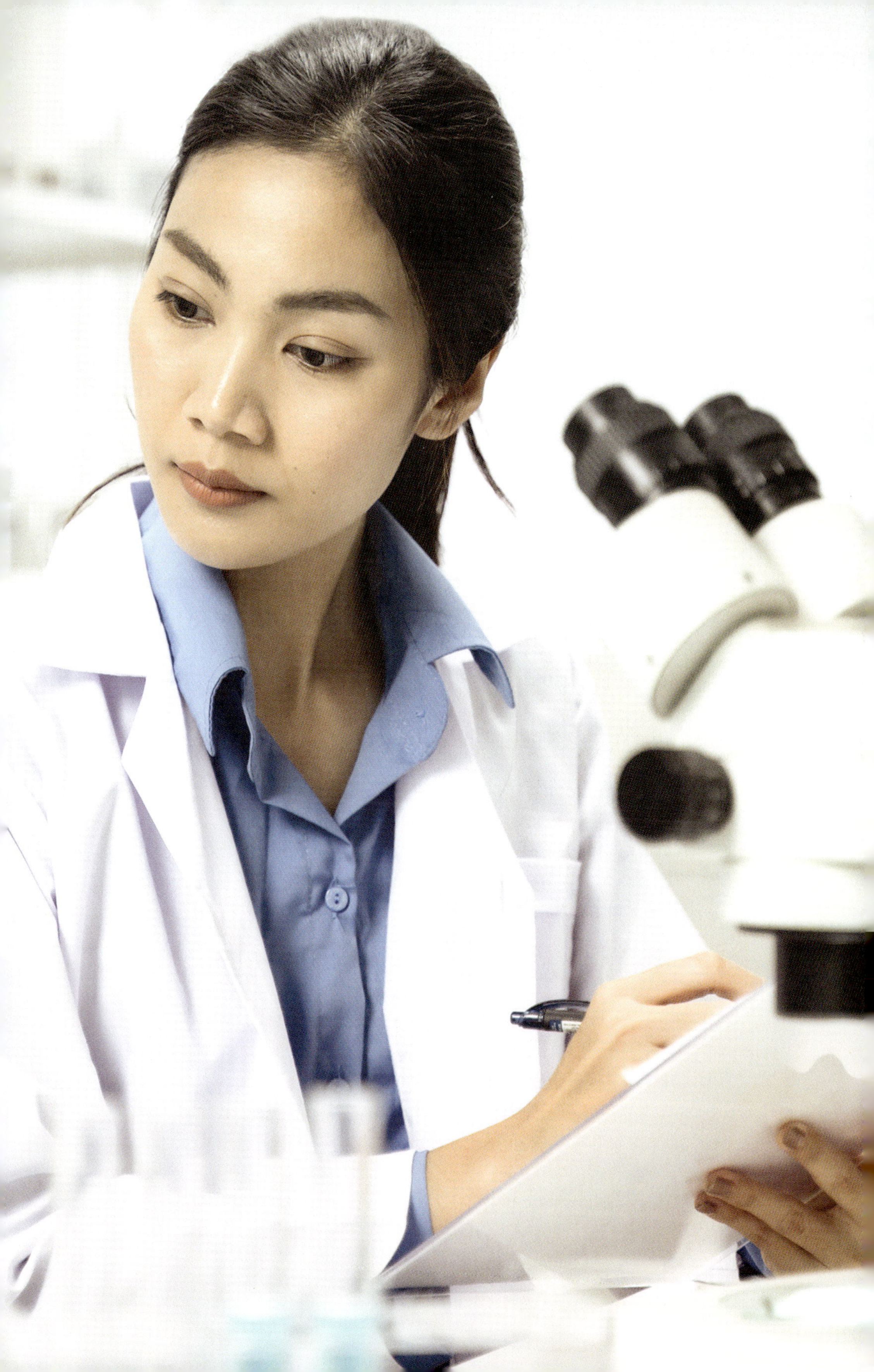

Nurses draw blood from patients all day. They also collect other fluids. This includes urine. They put the fluids in carefully marked containers. Then they send the containers through a tube delivery system. The samples arrive in the lab with a *whoosh*.

Conner picks up the vials. Then she becomes a detective. She tests the fluids. The results help doctors decide what is wrong with each patient.

Conner runs many different tests. Each requires specific tools or machines. She tests blood for sugar levels. She checks it for infections. She tests urine for protein. She uses a microscope to check for **parasites**.

CLTs must pay close attention to their work. Each test must be done with the

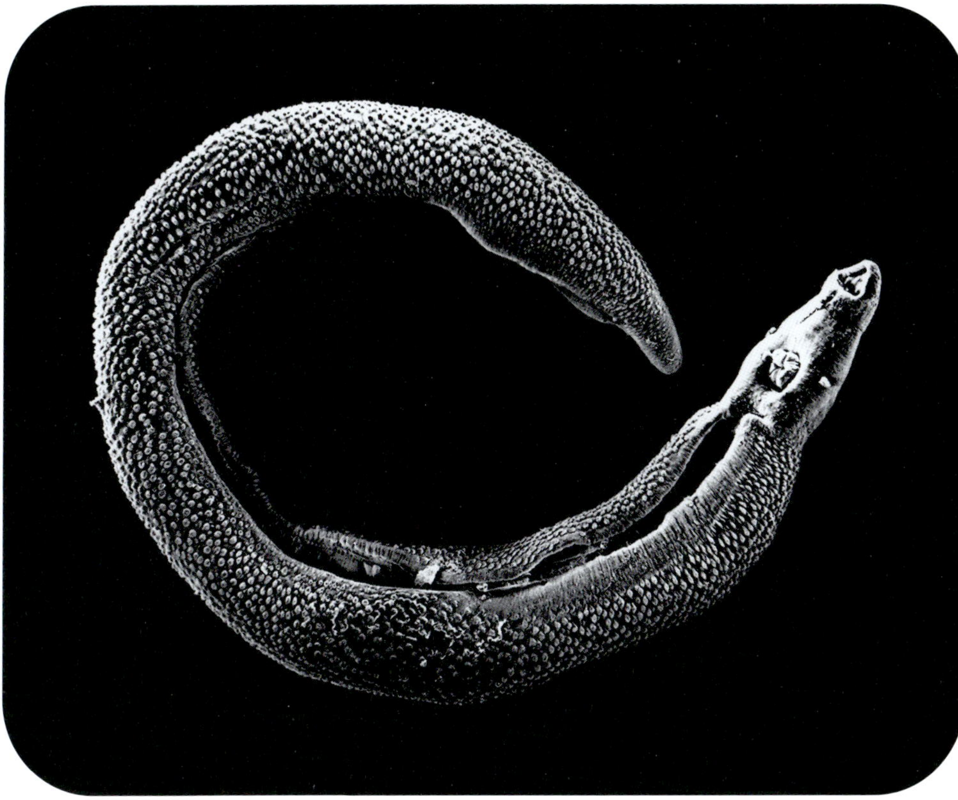

Some parasites, such as *Schistosoma*, can live in humans. Their eggs can be detected through urine and feces analyses.

proper machines. Each test also needs specific chemicals.

Conner uses **pipettes** to pick up small amounts of fluid for testing. She uses special scales to weigh tiny amounts of chemicals. She adds them to the fluids. When her tests are done, the results

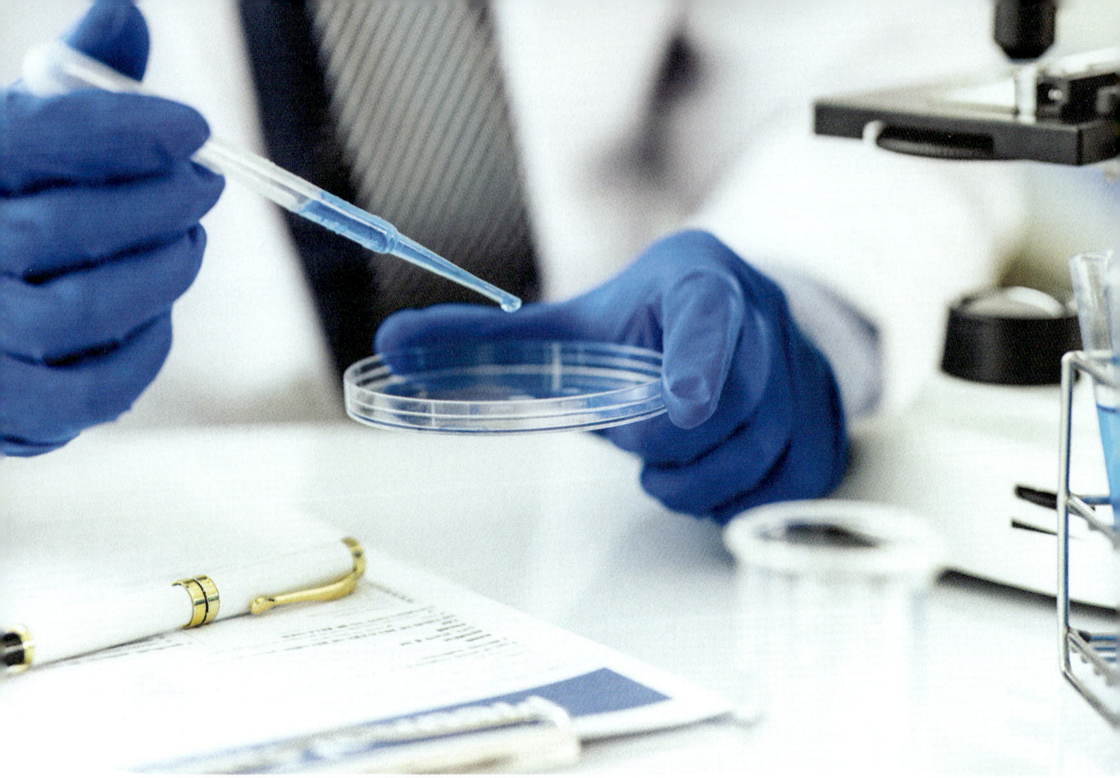

Pipettes can be made out of glass, plastic, or other materials.

go straight to the doctors. Doctors then figure out the best way to help each patient. Conner's work will help make patients healthy.

WHAT IS A CLINICAL LABORATORY TECHNICIAN?

Patients rarely see CLTs. But they play important roles in health care settings.

A CLT runs tests to help doctors figure out what is making a patient sick. They perform tests on bodily fluids. They also test **tissue** from patients' organs.

CLTs must know how to use many types of testing machines. They must also know how to fix these machines. They must be able to measure and record tiny amounts of fluids. CLTs must do their jobs carefully. Their tests can save lives.

CHAPTER ONE

WHAT DOES A CLINICAL LABORATORY TECHNICIAN DO?

CLTs have very important jobs. They perform many kinds of tests to identify and treat diseases. They run tests on fluids. They test poop and tissue. These tests can show why a patient is sick. Doctors and nurses look at the results of these tests. They use the results to figure out the best way to help their patients.

Most CLTs work in hospitals or labs. They work with many different test machines.

CLTs sometimes work alongside doctors and specialists to decide on a patient's treatment.

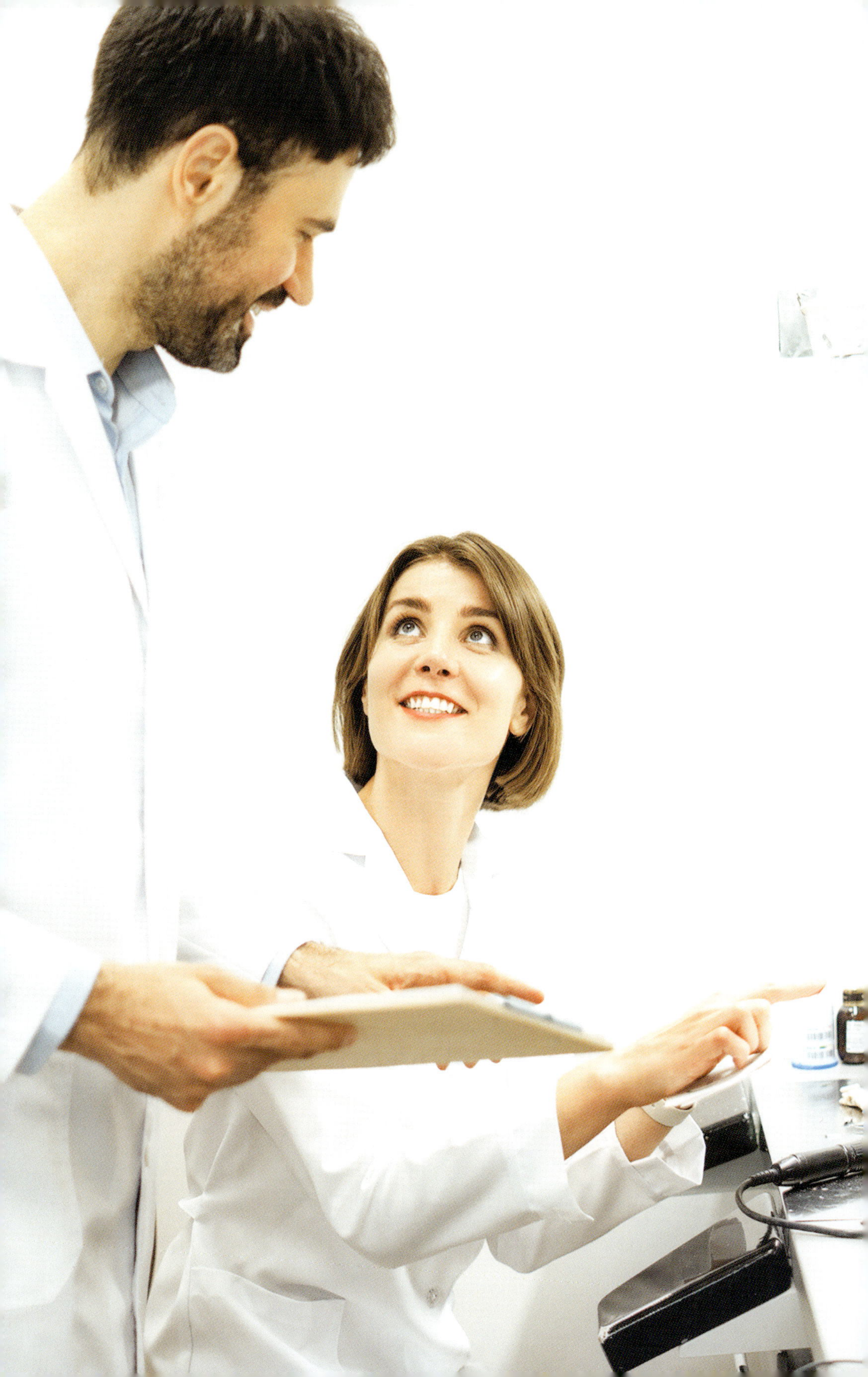

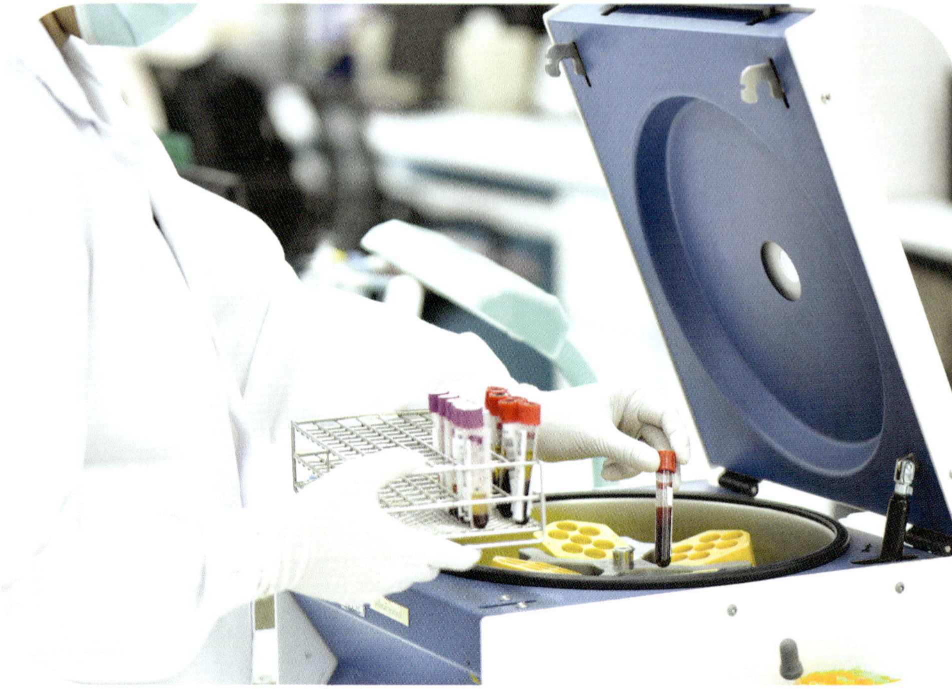

Some centrifuges keep samples refrigerated as they spin.

A CLT needs to know how to use the machines. They must also know how to take care of the machines. This is called maintenance. It keeps the machines running smoothly.

TECHNOLOGY AND TOOLS

CLTs perform different tests with different machines. This means CLTs must be familiar with many different machines. One machine CLTs often use is a centrifuge.

A centrifuge is a machine that spins tubes around. The tubes are filled with fluids. Some centrifuges can spin tubes thousands of times per minute. The fast spinning separates the fluids into different parts. Clinical laboratory technicians look at these different parts to detect problems and diseases.

Layers of Blood

Blood spun in a centrifuge separates into different parts. The heaviest layer has red blood cells. It goes to the bottom. A thin layer called the buffy coat is next. It contains white blood cells and platelets. At the top is a liquid called plasma. CLTs sample and test each part.

Another common tool is a microscope. This tool helps CLTs see things that are very small. Some make objects look 1,000 times bigger. Technicians can then look closely at samples.

Microscopes help CLTs see tiny germs. They can look at poop samples and see tapeworm eggs. Or they might see dangerous parasites. This can help explain why someone is sick.

A CLT must prepare a sample of what they are testing before using a microscope. They place a sample on a thin piece of glass. This is called a microscope slide. A sample could be a drop of blood. Or it could be a bit of tissue. Sometimes another chemical is placed on the slide, too. This helps the sample show up better.

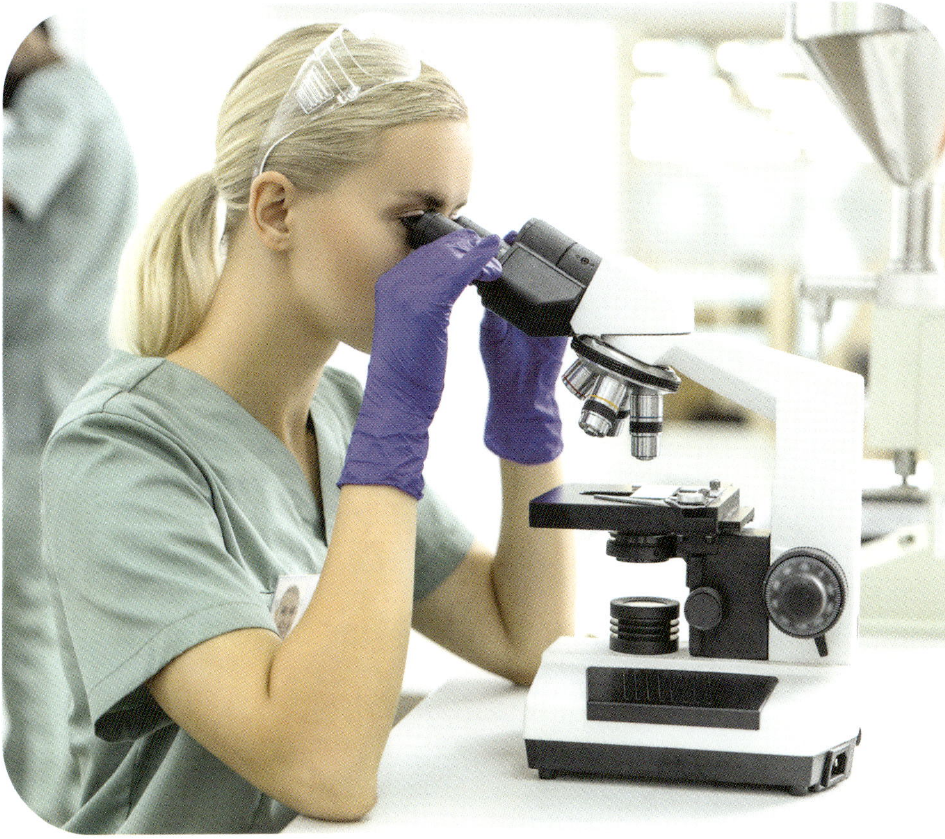

Laboratory microscopes can cost anywhere from $1,000 to more than $20,000.

Another piece of glass may then be placed on top. This is called a cover slip.

The CLT then looks through the microscope's eyepiece. They adjust the microscope. Microscopes usually have several **lenses**. Each magnifies a different amount. The CLT adjusts the microscope until the picture is clear. Then they look for anything unusual in the sample.

CLTs also use spectrophotometers. These tools shine light through liquids. Then they measure the amount of light that passes through the liquid. This can determine the amount of sugar or iron in a patient's blood. It can also test urine for drugs or infections.

Another important machine is the hematology analyzer. This machine measures parts of a person's blood. Looking at these parts can help doctors spot infections. It can also help doctors spot cancer.

Coagulation analyzers also test blood. These machines determine whether a person's blood is sticking together properly.

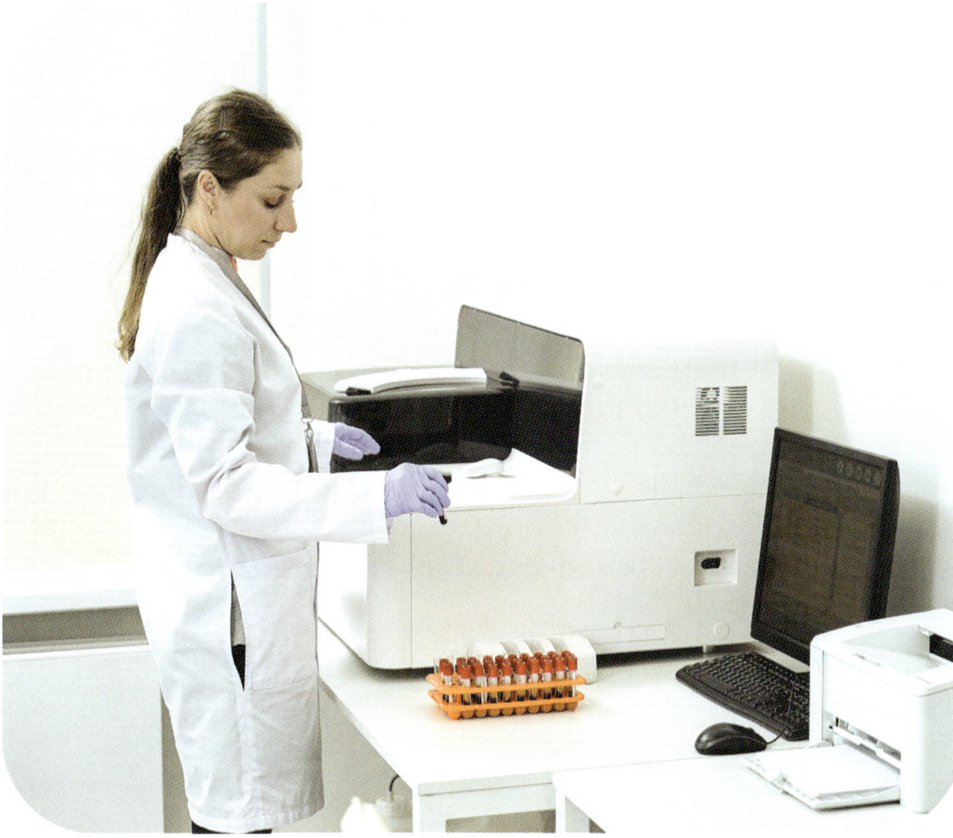

Hematology analyzers can detect blood disorders such as anemia and leukemia.

This is called clotting. Clotting stops people from bleeding too much when they get wounds.

Blood gas analyzers also perform blood tests. These machines use electricity to check the levels of oxygen and carbon dioxide in a person's blood. This can determine if a person's lungs are working well. Low oxygen levels may mean a person is sick. They may have a lung disease. Blood gas analyzers also measure the pH of blood. This is how acidic something is.

Urine tests that use colored strips are called urine dipstick tests.

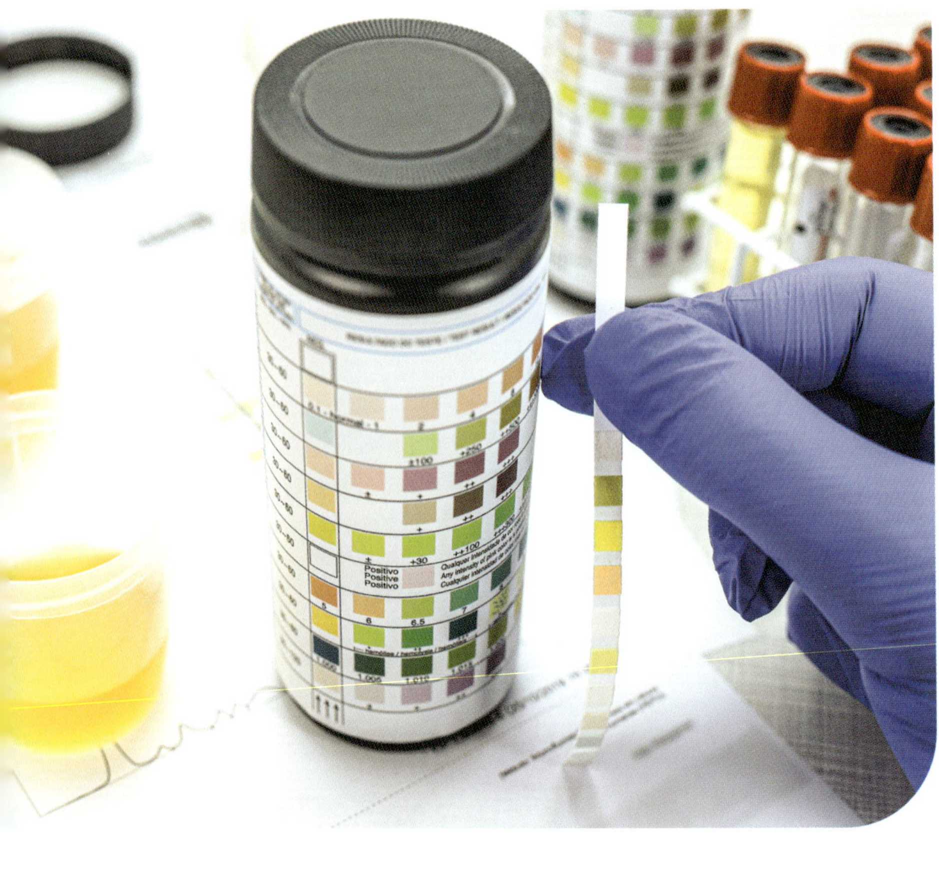

Sometimes CLTs test urine. This can be done in several ways. Some tests use plastic strips. These are dipped in urine. The strips then change colors. The colors on each strip tell the CLT if certain chemicals are present.

Urine tests can check for blood in a person's pee. They can also test for glucose or ketones. People with diabetes may have these chemicals in their urine. People with heart or kidney problems might have protein in their urine.

A CLT may also use a urine analyzer machine. This machine can perform urine tests automatically. It still uses plastic strips. But it can test hundreds of samples each hour. It also interprets test results. This is faster than testing urine manually.

CLTs use many more machines. Some test for diseases. Others help CLTs measure fluids. Still others help them mix chemicals. Each tool helps CLTs take care of patients.

ATTENTION TO DETAIL

Knowing how to use testing equipment is not a CLT's only job. CLTs are also responsible for making sure they have enough chemicals and supplies. One of the first things Kim Conner does every day is check her supplies. She makes sure she has test tubes. She also needs pipettes. CLTs must also have microscope slides. Connor makes sure she has enough chemicals to run tests in the different machines.

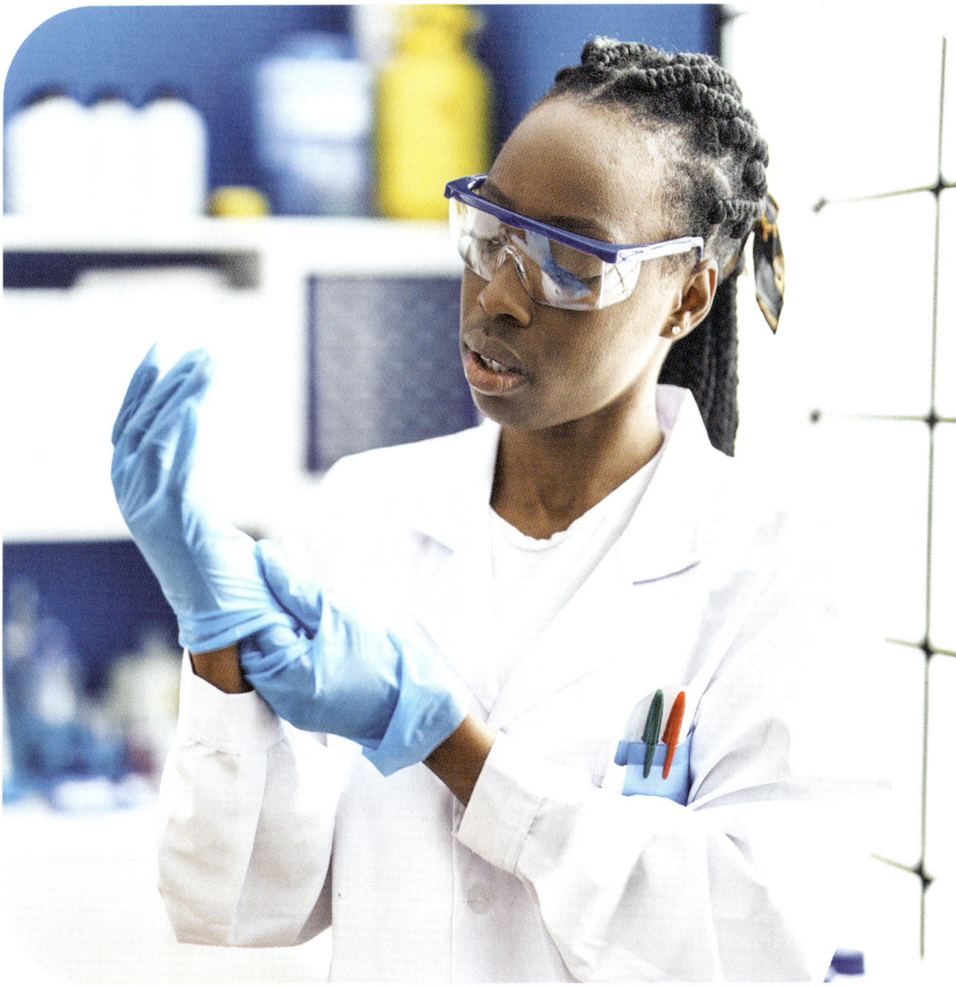

Safety equipment such as gloves and safety glasses is often called personal protective equipment, or PPE.

Other supplies keep CLTs safe. CLTs should never directly touch samples. This could make them sick. So they must have safety equipment. This equipment includes gloves. It also includes safety glasses. It is

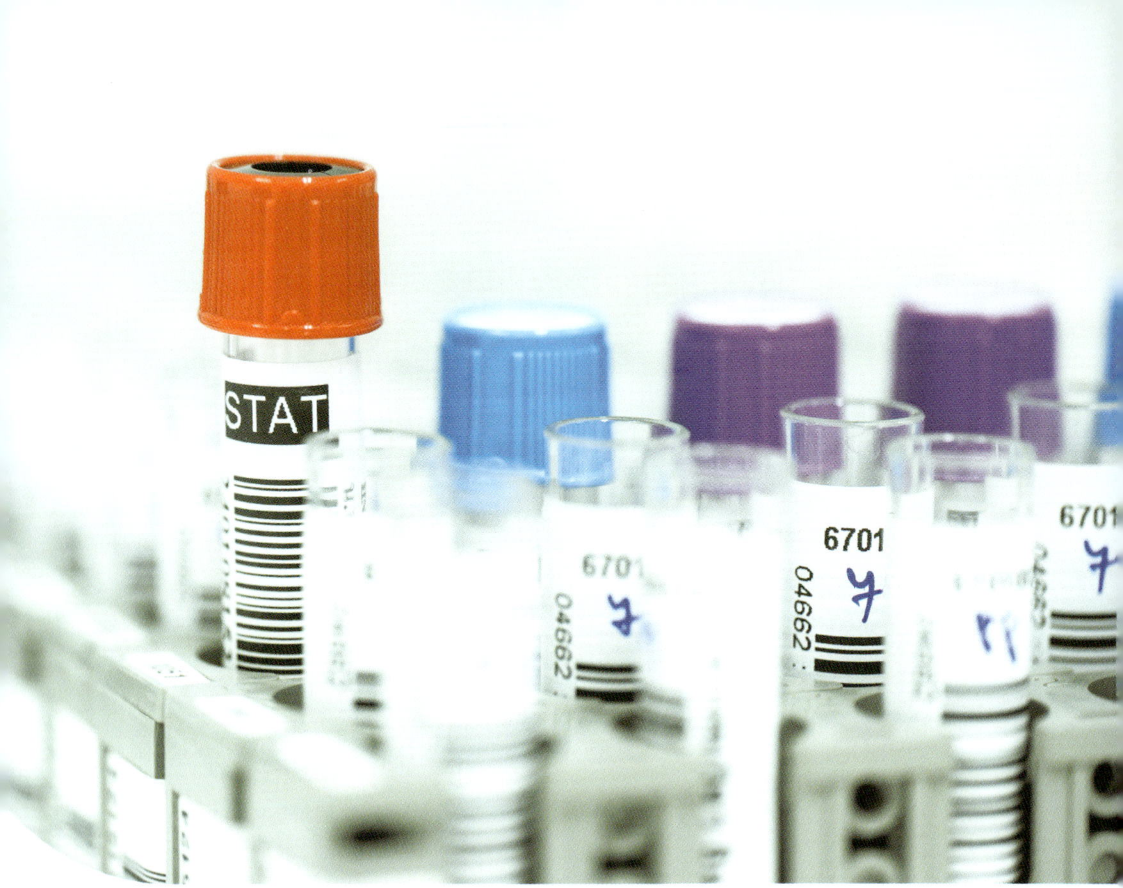

All samples must be carefully labeled and handled. Otherwise they may be mixed up, leading to a diagnosis being given to the wrong patient.

important to have everything ready before starting the day.

The next step is to make sure all the machines are working. CLTs run simple tests. They see if the machines work. They make sure they are clean. They check that the scales are set to zero.

CLTs then spend their days running tests. Each test is important to a patient. Each test helps a doctor decide how to make their patient better.

It is very important to make sure each test result goes to the correct patient. CLTs must carefully read the labels on each test tube. They put this information into their computer systems. They must know how to use the computer systems anywhere they work. The information is sent to doctors. Sometimes CLTs have discussions with doctors about the test results.

CLTs spend all day running tests. Then they clean up their workspaces. They check the levels of their supplies. They order more if needed. They might turn off the machines. But labs in big hospitals never close.

The machines keep running. Night workers come in to take the daytime CLTs' places.

DETECTIVE WORK

"Many people consider us medical detectives," says Vicki Freeman. She teaches CLTs at a college. She explains why CLTs are important, saying, "The people we educate are the ones who work in the labs processing **specimens** that come to them from patients. They perform the tests that go back to **physicians**, allowing them to make decisions on how to treat patients."[2]

The Centers for Disease Control and Prevention (CDC) is a US government agency. It works to improve public health. Part of this includes researching how US hospitals work.

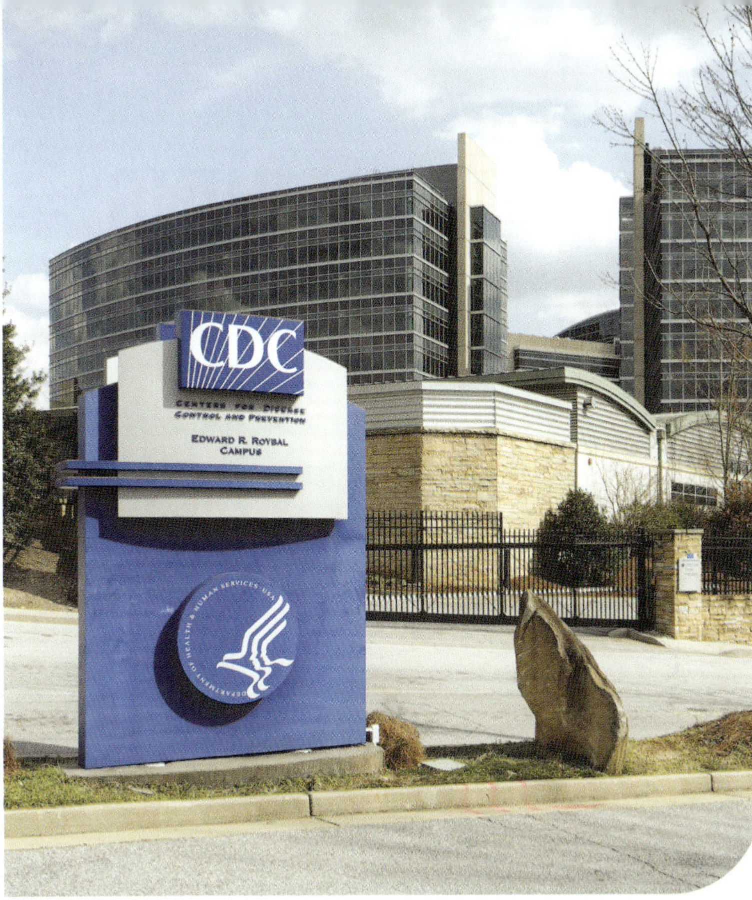

The CDC is headquartered in Atlanta, Georgia.

The CDC estimates that 70 percent of medical decisions depend on laboratory tests. More than 14 billion tests are done each year. This makes CLTs important parts of the health care system. It also means their work helps millions of people stay healthy.

CHAPTER TWO

WHAT TRAINING DO CLINICAL LABORATORY TECHNICIANS NEED?

Learning to be a CLT is challenging. But it is also fun. CLTs must be educated. They must graduate from high school. This is where they learn basic skills in math. They also learn science skills. They may take biology and chemistry.

These basic skills are important for a person's next level of training. People who want to be CLTs must go to college. Some take 2-year programs. They get

High school students who like math and science may enjoy careers as CLTs.

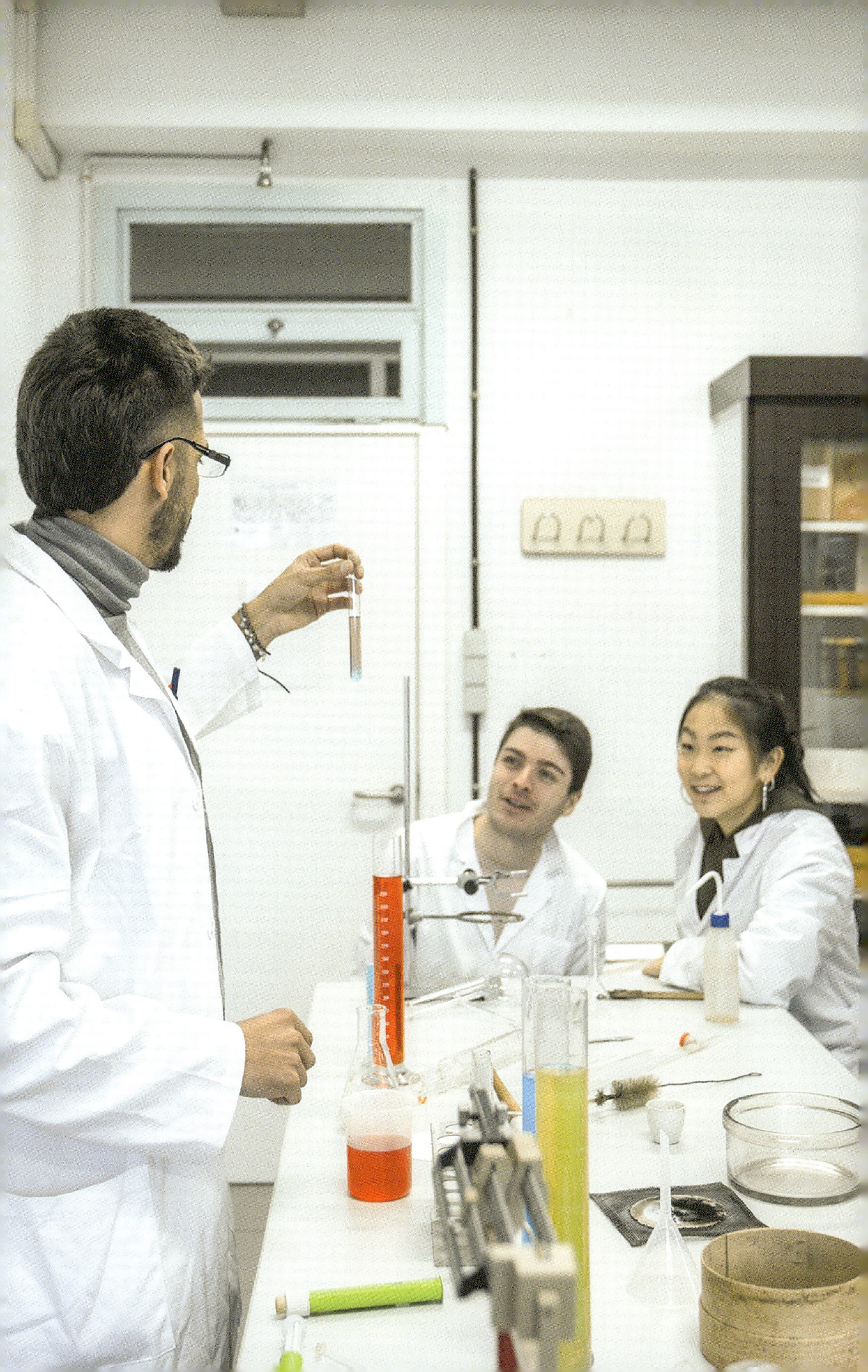

associate degrees. This allows them to become medical laboratory technicians (MLTs). An MLT is a type of CLT.

Some students study for 4 years. These students graduate with bachelor's degrees. They can be certified as medical laboratory scientists (MLSs). An MLS is another type of CLT. But MLSs are more advanced than MLTs. MLSs can get higher positions in their workplaces. They can become **supervisors**. They may also become teachers.

LEVELS OF TRAINING

CLTs must take exams after graduating. Those who pass the tests get certifications. A certification proves that a person has certain skills. CLT certifications come

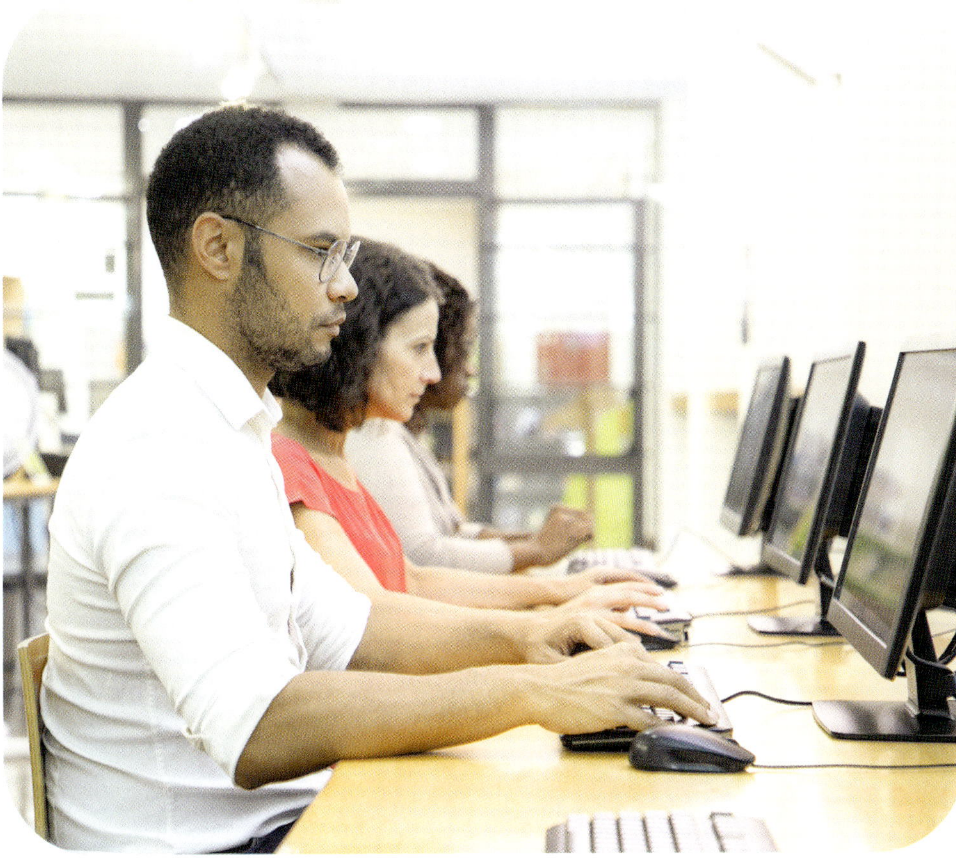

The American Society for Clinical Pathology offers certificate exams for MLSs, MLTs, and a wide range of specialists.

from several organizations. One such organization is the American Society for Clinical Pathology. This organization certifies both MLTs and MLSs.

The American Association of Bioanalysts also certifies CLTs. People who have

2-year degrees can be certified by this organization. Those who pass

CLTs weigh chemicals using sensitive scales called analytical balances.

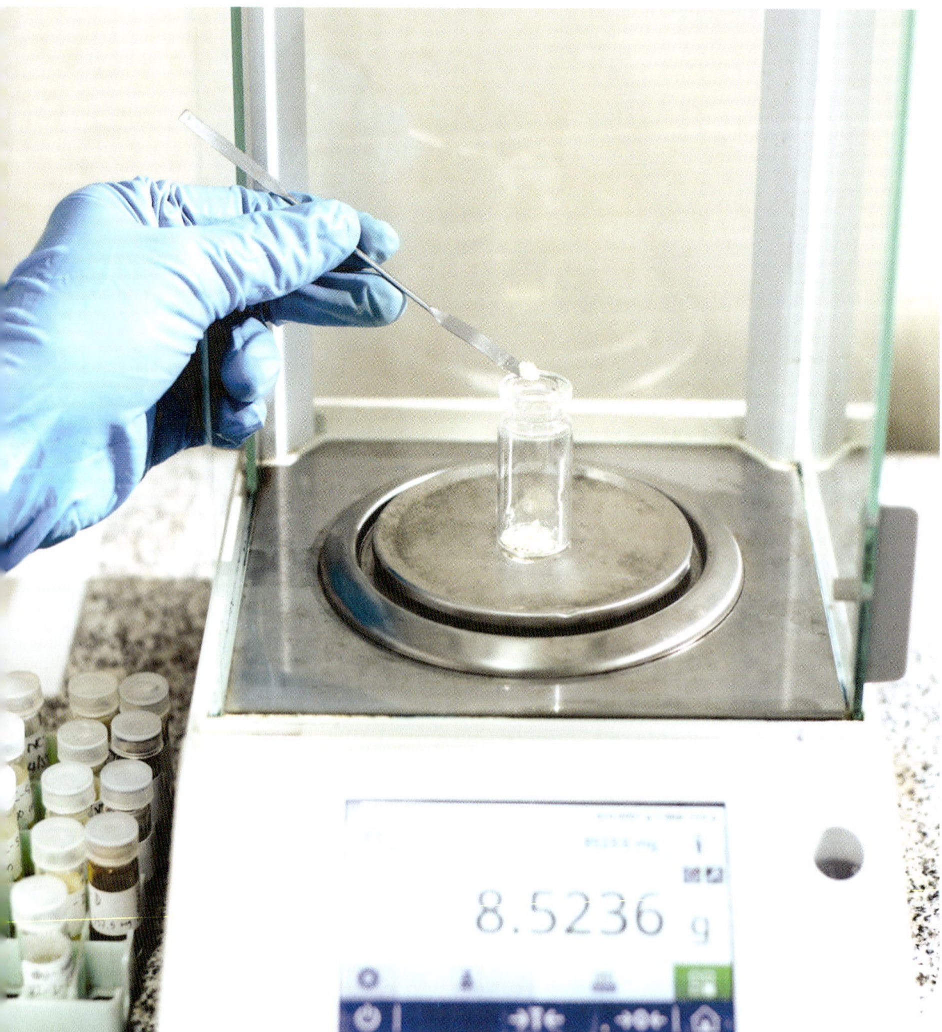

the tests earn the title of medical laboratory technologist. This certification is somewhere between an MLT and an MLS.

SCHOOLWORK AND LABORATORIES

Training to be a CLT is done in three steps. Students first go to lectures. They learn about the machines. They learn how to run tests. They also learn about science. Some courses are about chemistry. Others focus on more specific topics. One such topic is blood. This is because blood is one of the most tested bodily fluids. Other courses might focus on parasites or viruses.

Students then practice using testing machines. College labs have a wide variety of these machines. They are usually smaller than the machines in actual labs. Kara Stamper teaches for a college medical laboratory technology program. She says, "Students learn to perform a lot of different types of testing in the clinical laboratory."[3] This prepares students for their future careers.

Students practice other CLT tasks. They learn to use pipettes to pick up tiny drops of fluid. They practice weighing and mixing chemicals. Students grow **cultures** to test for infections. They learn to count cells.

Students eventually start clinical rotations. This is when students go to real labs. They are taught by actual CLTs. They get to see what life is like in the career. They even get to do real CLT work. They run the same tests they learned in their college labs.

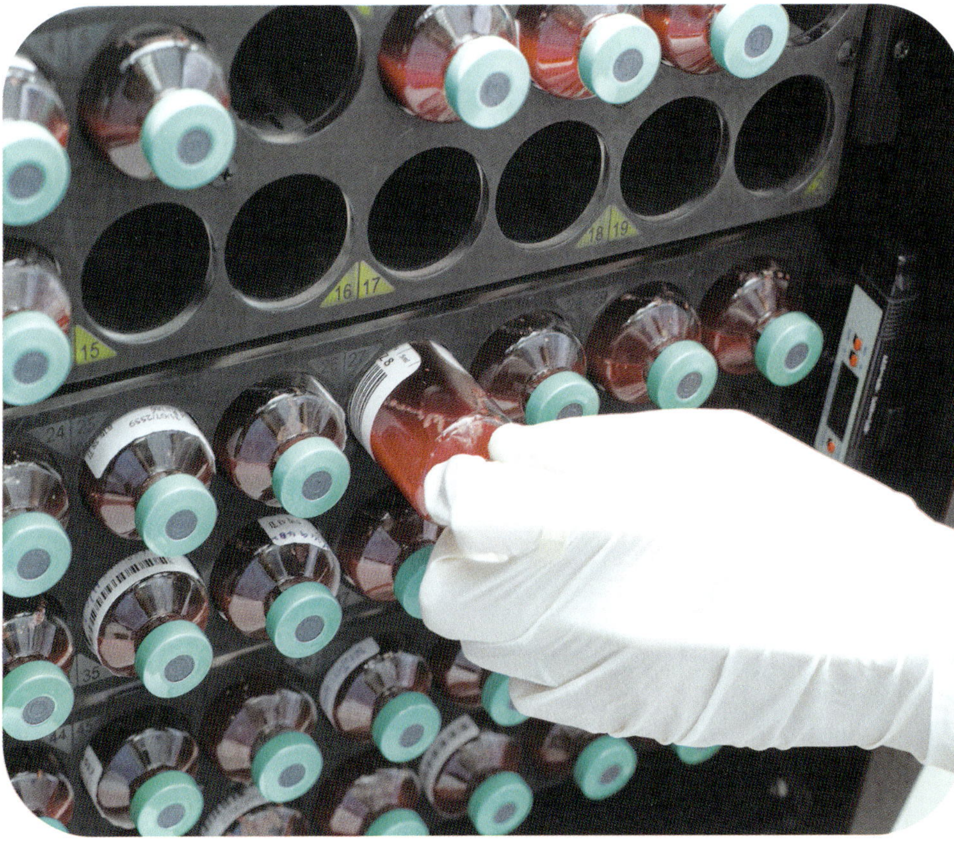

Incubators keep blood cultures warm to allow bacteria and fungi to grow.

But this time they are testing samples from actual patients. And their work is supervised by a professional.

SPECIAL CERTIFICATIONS

Some CLTs specialize. This means a CLT chooses one subject. Then they become

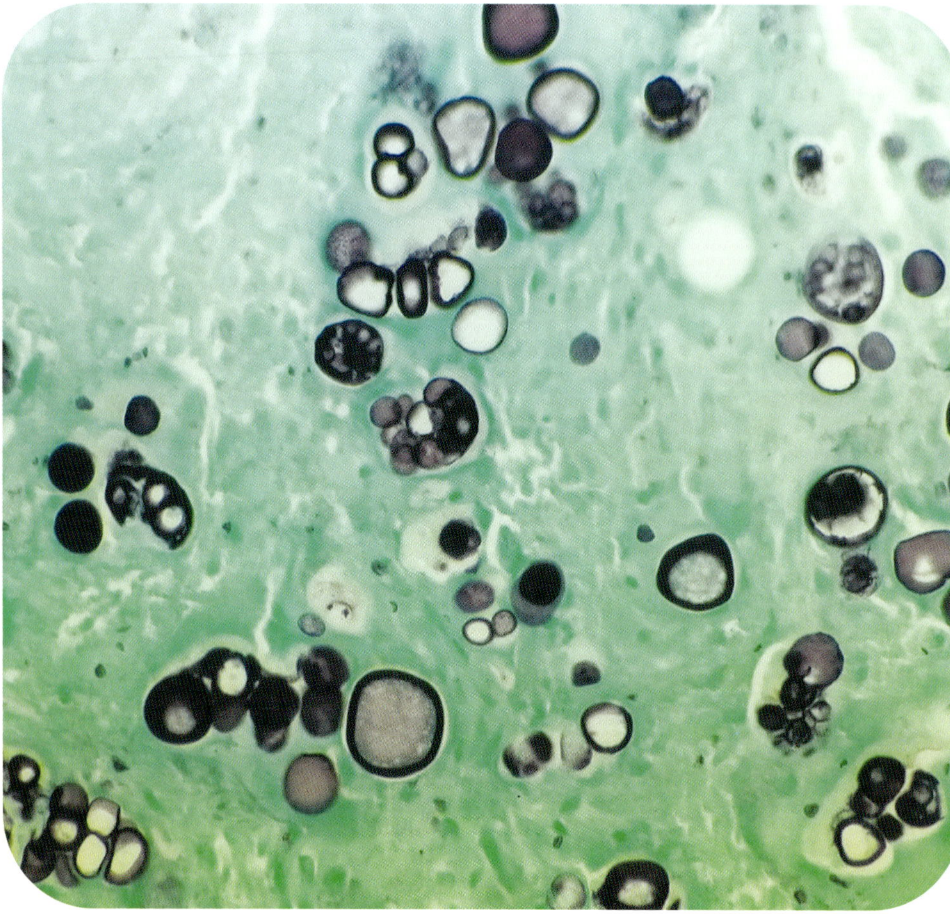

The fungus *Coccidioides* causes valley fever, a disease that can infect a person's lungs.

an expert in that area. This requires more in-depth study.

One area CLTs can specialize in is microbiology. Faezeh Zahedi is a CLT. She specializes in microbiology. She says, "Microbiology is the study of microorganisms."[4] These are tiny living things. They include bacteria.

Microbiology CLTs learn a lot about bacteria. They also learn about fungi. They are experts at growing cultures. It is their job to figure out what germs are causing infections. They also learn which medicines fight each infection.

Other CLTs might specialize in clinical chemistry. These CLTs learn about

Feeding Diseases

Laboratory technicians grow cultures to learn about diseases. They take a small sample of germs. Then they give the germs food. They let the germs grow in small dishes called petri dishes. The germs grow into large colonies. This gives the technicians plenty of germs to study.

human organs. They know how to test that the organs are working correctly. A clinical chemistry CLT may test a person's cholesterol to check for heart disease. They test oxygen levels in blood to see how the lungs are working.

Hematology is another specialty. It deals with the study of blood. A hematology CLT may look at blood through a microscope. They see if a person has enough red blood cells. They check for parasites living in the blood. They count white blood cells to search for indications of infection. They also do many other tests.

Other specialties include immunology and histotechnology. Immunology is the study of how the body fights off germs. Immunologists specialize in infections.

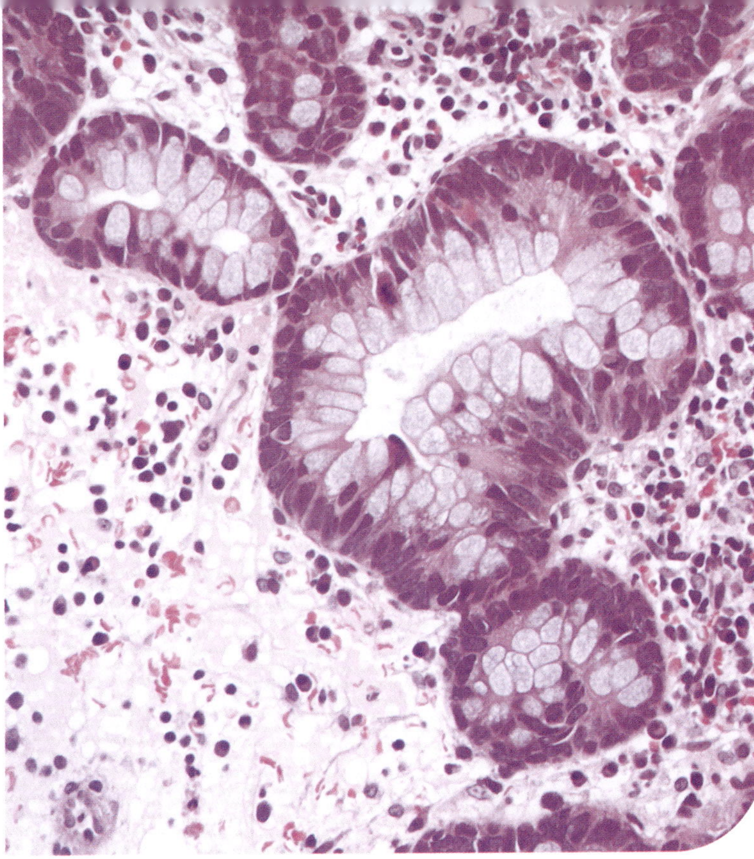

Histotechnologists may use microscopes to look for cancer cells in lung tissue.

Histotechnologists look at tiny slices of tissue. They look for signs of diseases such as cancer.

CHAPTER THREE

WHAT IS LIFE LIKE AS A CLINICAL LABORATORY TECHNICIAN?

A CLT can have a range of schedules. Some CLTs have day shifts. They might work from 8:00 a.m. to 4:00 p.m. This is when many clinics are open. Others work overnight. They may work at testing facilities. Hospitals also often have overnight workers. But there are usually fewer night workers than day workers.

The hours worked in a day can also vary. Day shift CLTs often work 8-hour days.

CLTs generally take turns working during holidays.

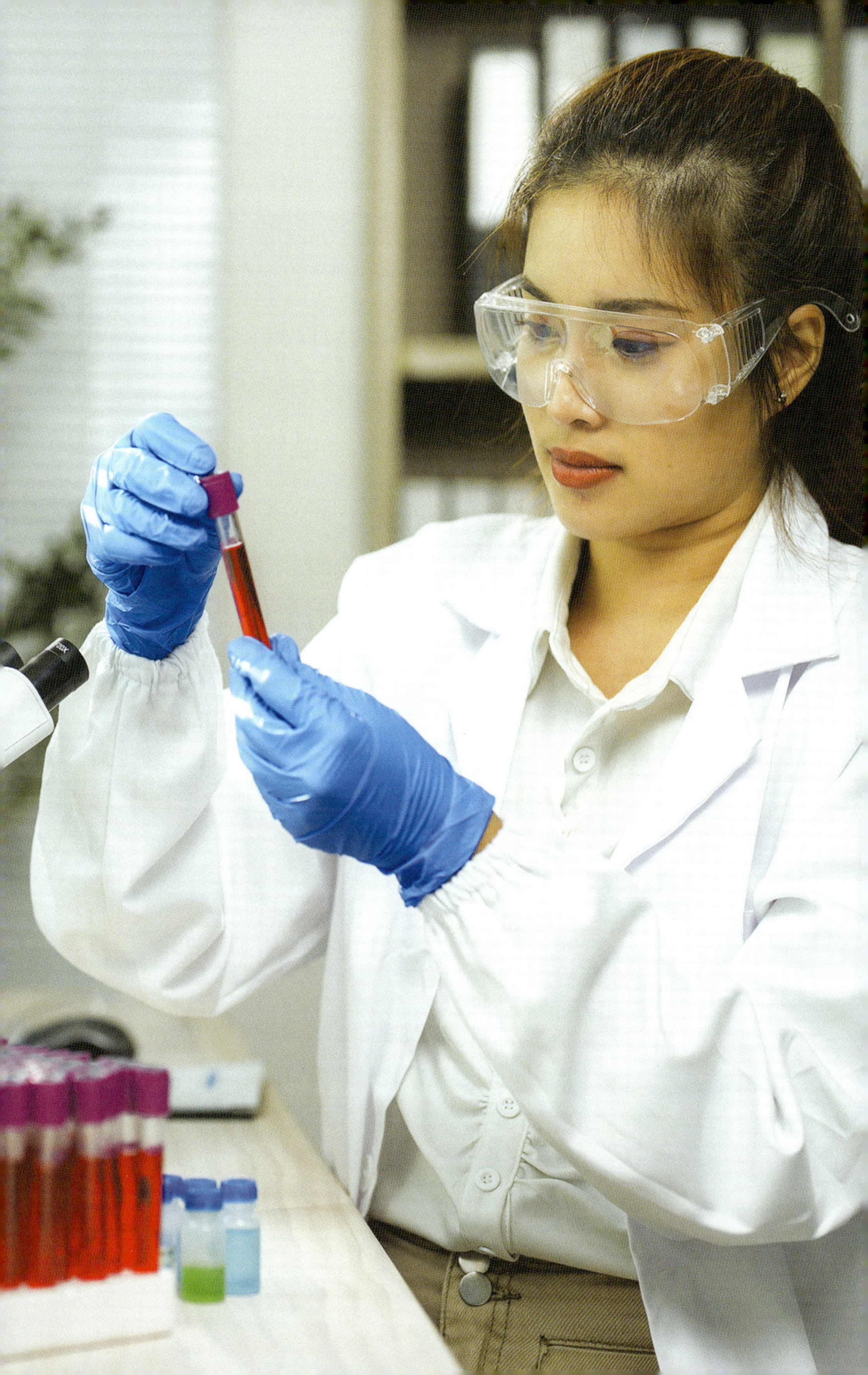

They work 5 days a week. These CLTs have usually been in the field for a while. Night shift workers tend to be newer. They often work 10- to 12-hour shifts. But they may work fewer days each week.

A CLT's hours depend on the facility at which they work. Their schedule also depends on the number of CLTs who

CLTs often work in team settings.

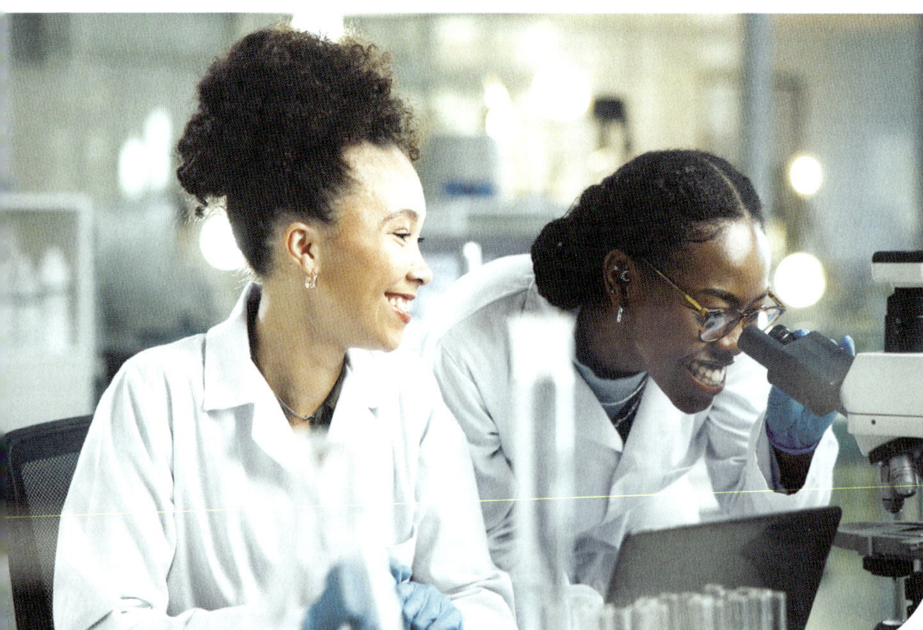

work with them. Small clinics may have only one or two CLTs. But large labs have many more. These places often have 40 or more CLTs.

THE WORKSPACE

Clinical laboratory technicians have unusual workplaces. Their workplaces are full of testing machines. There are refrigerators full of chemicals. Other refrigerators contain blood and other specimens. Work areas are filled with test tubes and other tools.

Only staff are allowed into labs. This means there are no patients allowed. Patients in big hospitals rarely meet with CLTs. Most CLTs work only with other technicians. But sometimes they discuss their results with doctors.

Smaller clinics may be different. CLTs at small clinics may collect samples from patients. These samples include blood and urine. They may also perform swab tests. These tests swab people's noses or throats. Then the CLTs can test for diseases. These diseases include COVID-19 and strep. But these tests are often done by other staff.

CLTs are often scheduled to work in certain sections of their labs each day. Different sections run different tests.

Taking Tiny Drops

Clinical laboratory technicians must measure tiny amounts of fluid. Pipettes make this possible. Pipettes come in many shapes and sizes. Some look like long needles. Some have gun-shaped handles on top. Fancy pipettes can suck up eight or more samples at a time.

One CLT might work in a section that tests blood. Another might work in an area testing urine. Another might be growing cultures.

CLTs spend their days running tests in their areas. But they may also help other CLTs. A CLT might have to cover a section while another takes a break.

WORKING WITH WEIRD THINGS

CLTs must be okay with seeing gross and weird things. They have to handle urine and blood. Sometimes they handle poop. They have to look at these samples under microscopes.

Sometimes CLTs see strange things under microscopes. They might see *Giardia* bugs in poop. These bugs look like triangular faces with two large eyes circled by eight strands of hair. CLTs might spot the African sleeping sickness parasite in blood. It looks like a blind, wiggling snake. Urine can contain shimmering crystals. One type of blood cancer looks like a wide-eyed owl. Seeing this wild combination of tiny forms is part of a CLT's job.

But weird and gross things are not just seen under the microscope. Lab refrigerators often contain body parts and organs. A long rectangular box in a cooler might hold a leg. Smaller boxes might hold thumbs and fingers. Seeing body parts can be an everyday occurrence. CLTs must be able to handle this. They must be able to touch these body parts. They are trained to test every part of the body.

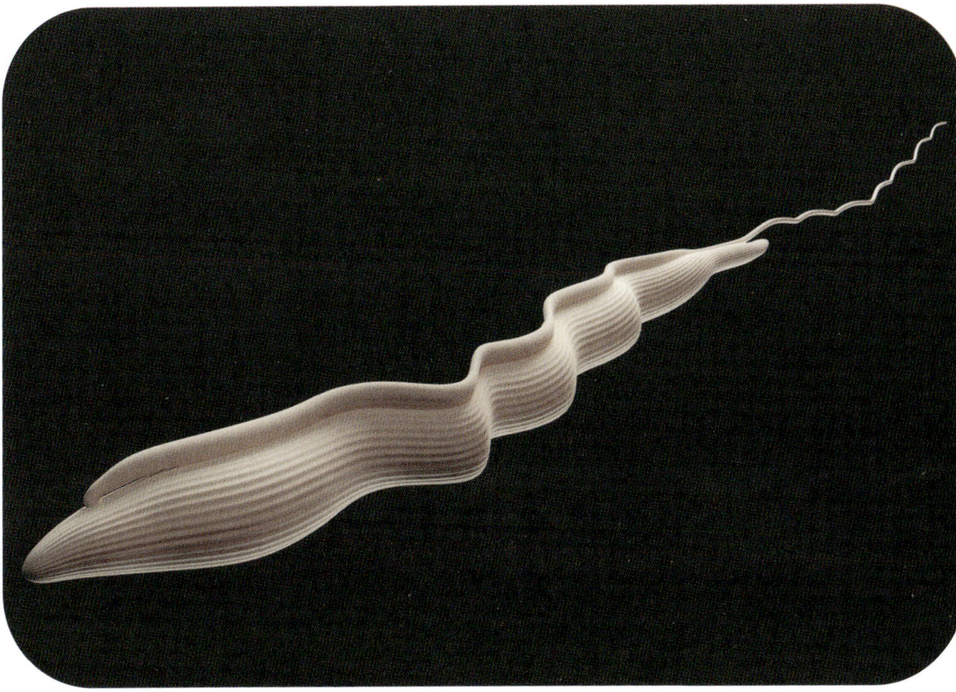

The African sleeping sickness parasite is spread through the bite of a fly.

Those who can handle this weird environment will find a fulfilling career. Faezeh Zahedi says:

> *We are basically like science detectives, trying to help the doctors to diagnose and choose the correct treatment for the patient. It makes me feel like I'm doing something good in this world.*[5]

CHAPTER FOUR

WHAT IS THE FUTURE FOR CLINICAL LABORATORY TECHNICIANS?

Clinical laboratory technicians have very important jobs. They give doctors the information to make good decisions. This means CLTs are needed around the world. They have a relatively easy time finding jobs.

The Bureau of Labor Statistics (BLS) is a US government agency. It collects information about different jobs. The BLS keeps track of where CLTs work. In 2024, it reported that 37 percent of CLTs worked

A career as a CLT is a good choice for someone who wants to make a difference.

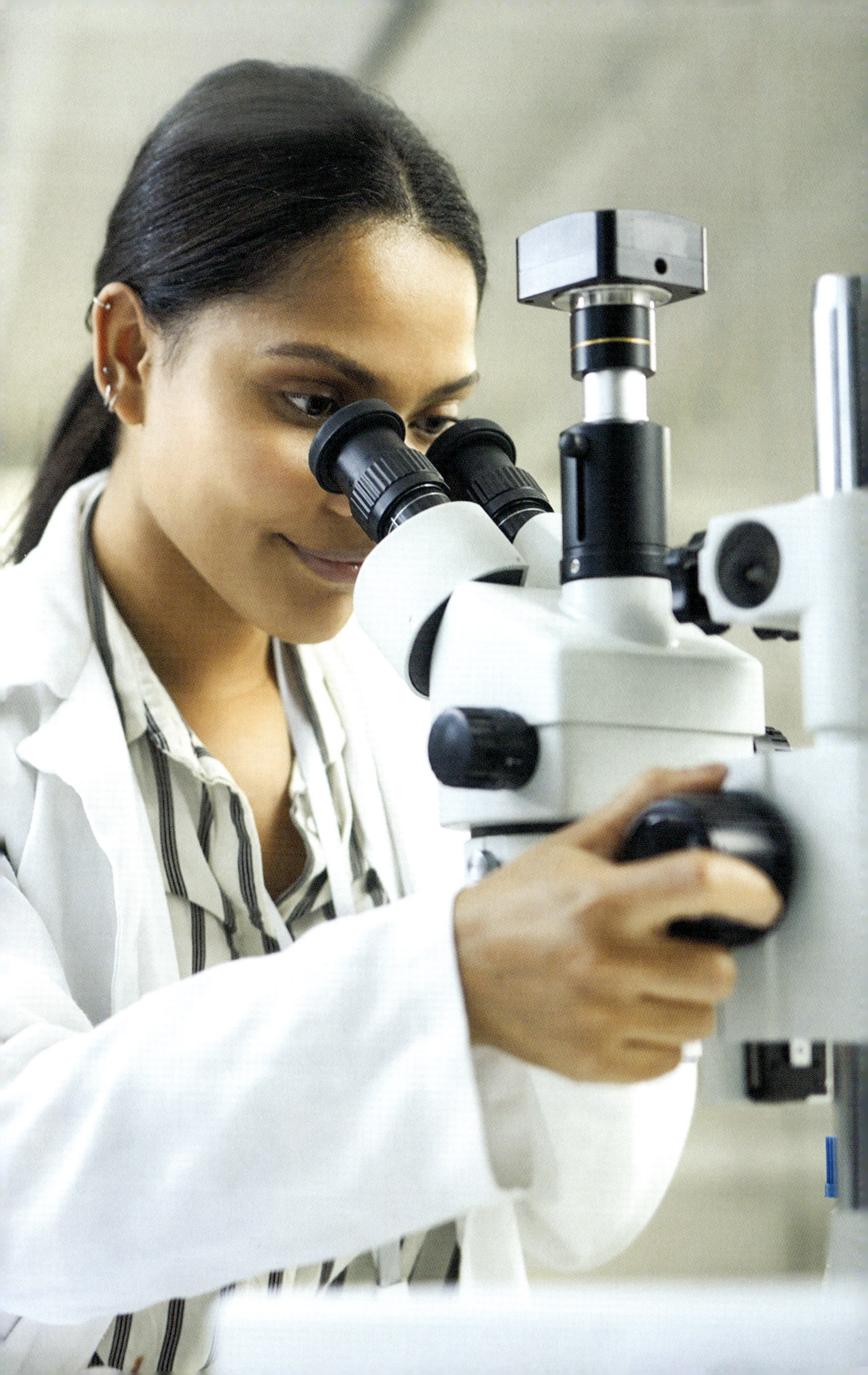

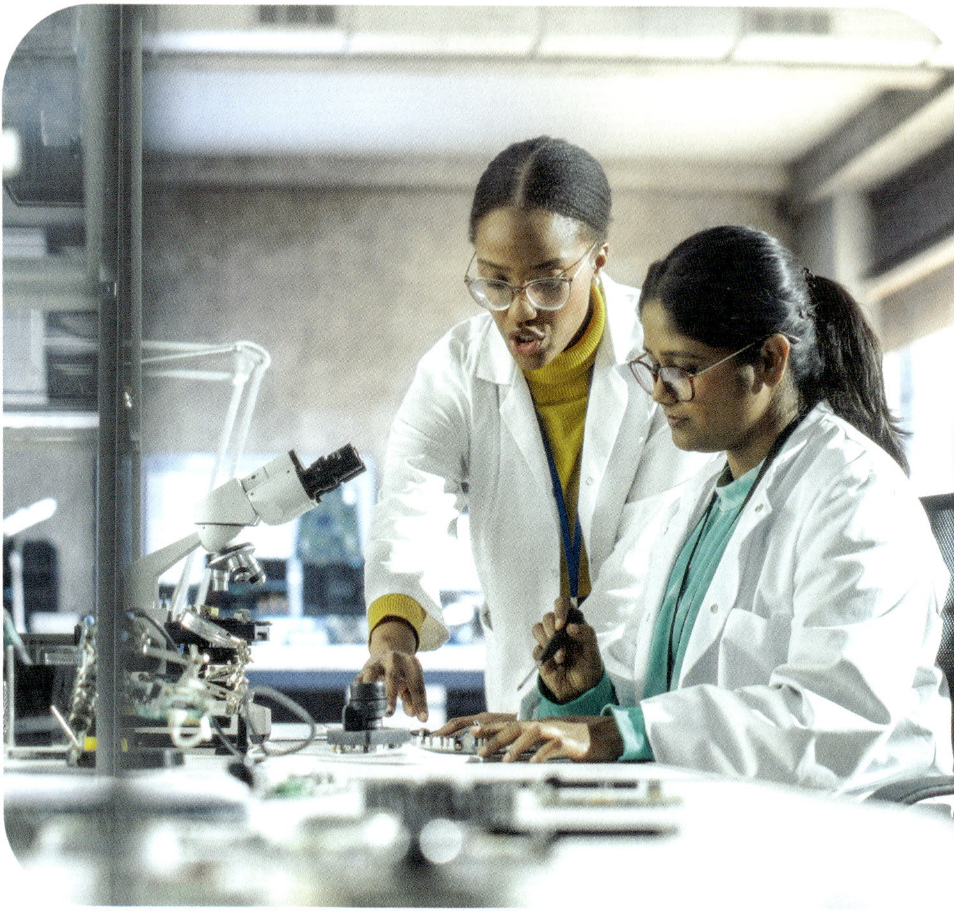

CLTs can go on to teach the next generation of lab workers.

in hospitals. Another 20 percent worked in labs. About 10 percent worked in clinics. CLTs also worked in education. Others worked for other health care services.

This wide variety of employers gives CLTs many options. They can work at many different places. They can work around the country.

The BLS also estimates how careers will grow. It predicted that CLT job opportunities would grow by 2 percent from 2024 to 2034. This means there will be about 22,600 CLT job openings each year. Many of these jobs come from workers who are retiring or leaving the field.

SALARIES

The BLS keeps track of how much money people in different careers can expect to make. In 2024, the median wage for CLTs was $61,890. This was a little lower than the nation's average. The average wage in 2024 was $65,470. But there are ways for CLTs to earn more.

AVERAGE CLT SALARY BY STATE IN 2023

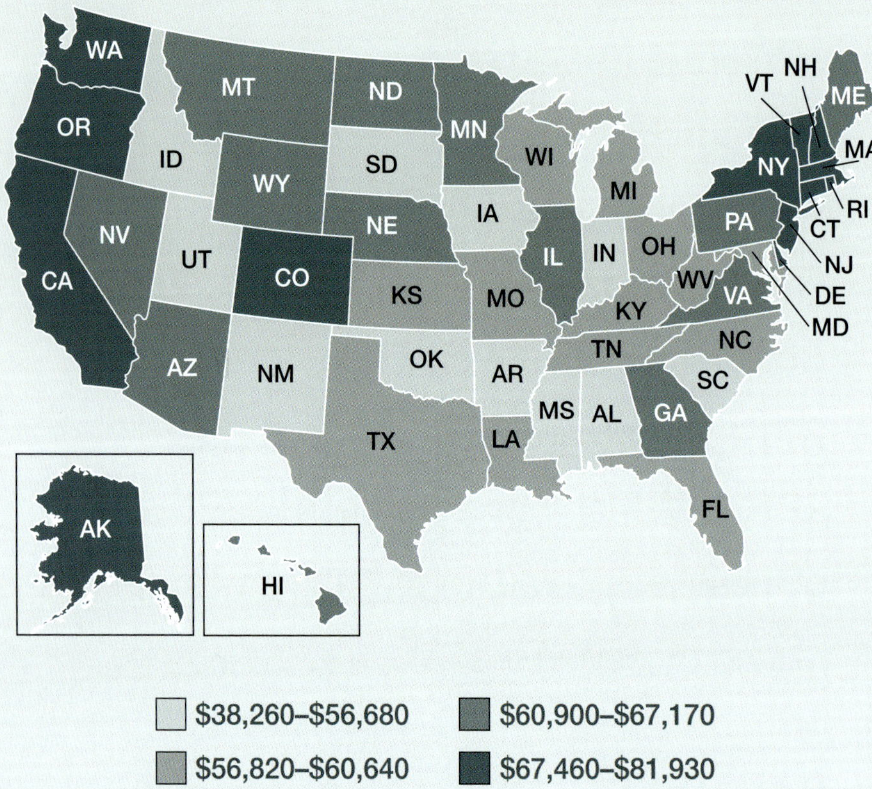

Source: "Geographic Profile for Clinical Laboratory Technologists and Technicians," US Bureau of Labor Statistics, *April 3, 2024. www.bls.gov.*

In 2023, the state with the highest average CLT salary was New York.

CLTs who work in hospitals earn more than those in other places. They earn an average of $66,650 each year. But the highest 10 percent earn much more. They make an average of nearly $100,000. Supervisors also earn more. CLT supervisors earn an average of $85,306.

It is also relatively easy for CLTs to get jobs. The job placement rate from 2-year programs is very high. Many colleges show a job placement rate of 100 percent for their graduates. Almost everyone who graduates can plan on quickly entering the field.

CLT Diversity

A variety of people work as clinical laboratory technicians. About 65 percent of workers are women. A little more than 50 percent are white. Nearly 18 percent are Hispanic or Latino. Roughly 13 percent are Asian. About 10 percent are Black. And about 8 percent of CLTs are part of the LGBT community.

AN INTELLIGENT FUTURE

CLTs might see big changes in their jobs. This is because some workplaces will start using artificial intelligence (AI). AI is a technology that can do complex tasks. It can process large amounts of information. It can write. It can spot patterns.

AI will not replace CLTs. But it will likely change how CLTs work. AI can sometimes be wrong. So CLTs will still have to program and supervise AI.

Aditi Sarkar is a CLT. She says, "As we look to the future, medical laboratory technology will continue to evolve."[6] AI will likely be part of many of these changes. It will affect everything from training to everyday lab work. These changes will

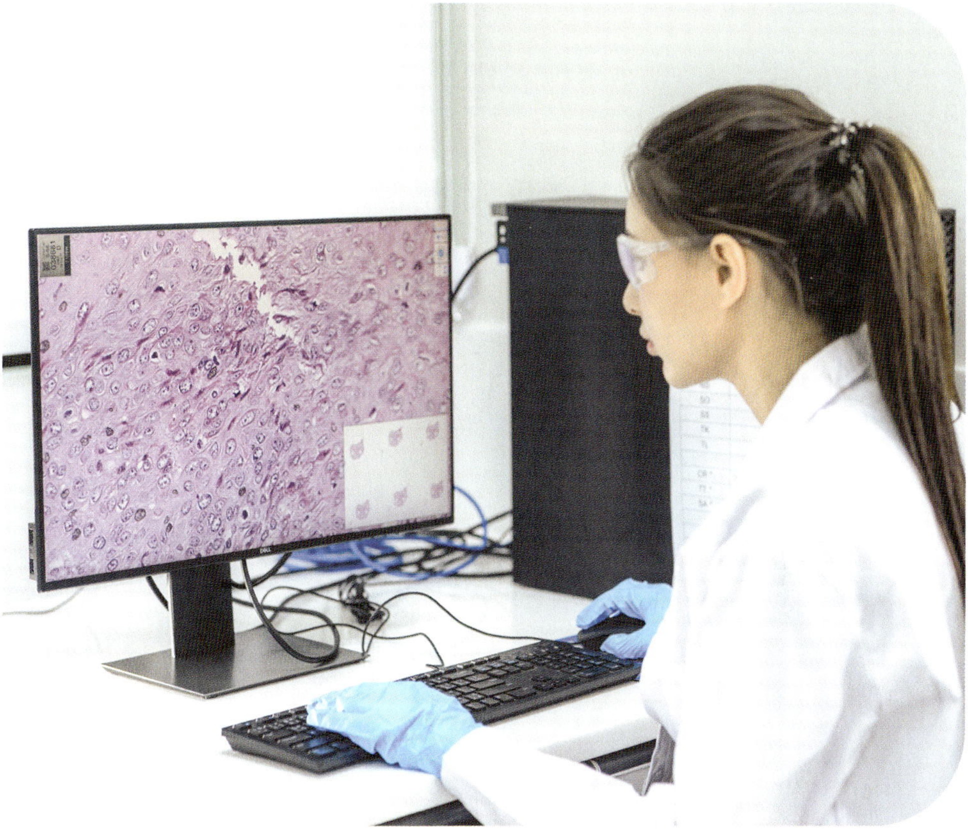

CLTs can use AI to test tissue samples for diseases, infections, and cancer.

help patients. AI can learn. This means it improves over time. AI may be able to suggest treatments for patients. It can detect errors. It may also be able to provide care for patients who are not near hospitals. New AI devices may be able to do tests away from labs.

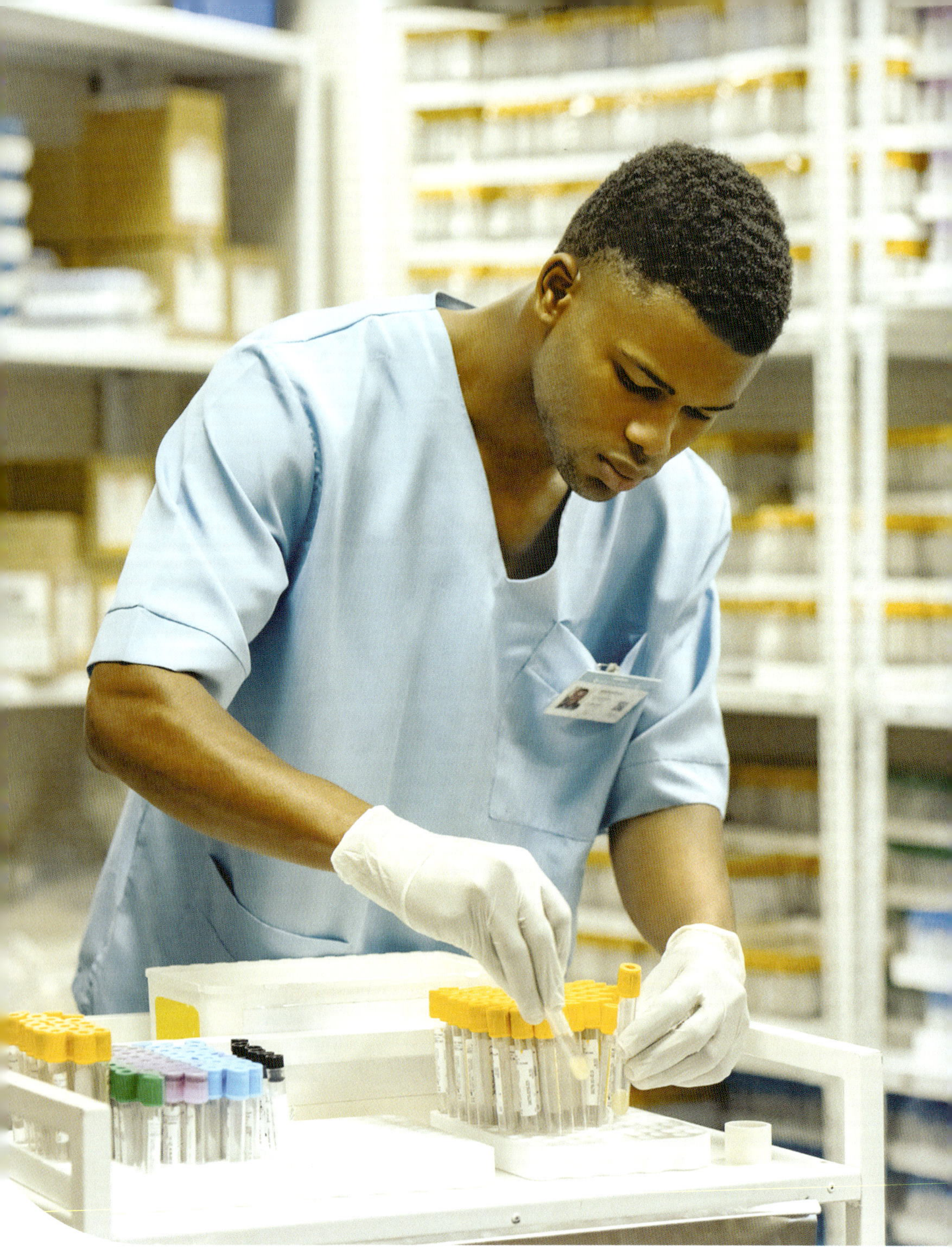

People who are fascinated by the human body may enjoy working as CLTs.

CLTs will continue to see their jobs change as technology evolves. But their roles will never stop being important. CLTs get to help people. And every day is a little different.

"If you love science, this field is incredible," says Kim Conner. "I can look at blood under a microscope and recognize cancer before anyone else knows—even the doctor. You never meet the patient, but you feel connected. We follow their progress and celebrate when results improve. It's rewarding, even without direct contact."[7]

GLOSSARY

cultures
bacteria or viruses that are grown in controlled settings

lenses
curved pieces of glass that magnify or focus images

parasites
organisms that live in other organisms and hurt their hosts

physicians
doctors

pipettes
tools used to measure and transfer tiny amounts of liquid

specimens
samples

supervisors
people who watch over another

tissue
material that makes up a living thing

SOURCE NOTES

INTRODUCTION: MEDICAL DETECTIVES

1. Kim Conner, Personal interview, September 29, 2025.

CHAPTER ONE: WHAT DOES A CLINICAL LABORATORY TECHNICIAN DO?

2. Quoted in Kurt Koopmann, "Laboratorians: Behind the Scenes Detectives," *Texas Medical Center*, August 4, 2017. www.tmc.edu.

CHAPTER TWO: WHAT TRAINING DO CLINICAL LABORATORY TECHNICIANS NEED?

3. Quoted in "Medical Laboratory Technology Program at Central Piedmont," *YouTube*, uploaded by Central Piedmont Community College, December 16, 2019. www.youtube.com.

4. Quoted in "A Day in the Life of a Medical Laboratory Technician," *YouTube*, uploaded by Tahatū Career Navigator, February 23, 2021. www.youtube.com.

CHAPTER THREE: WHAT IS LIFE LIKE AS A CLINICAL LABORATORY TECHNICIAN?

5. Quoted in "A Day in the Life of a Medical Laboratory Technician."

CHAPTER FOUR: WHAT IS THE FUTURE FOR CLINICAL LABORATORY TECHNICIANS?

6. Aditi Sarkar, "Embracing Innovation: Transformative Trends in the Laboratory," *American Society for Clinical Laboratory Science* 38, no. 3, June 2024. https://ascls.org.

7. Kim Conner, Personal interview, September 29, 2025.

FOR FURTHER RESEARCH

BOOKS

Knowledge Encyclopedia: Human Body. Wonder House Books, 2022.

Marie-Therese Miller, *Jobs in Health Care*. Abdo Publishing, 2024.

Sarina Peterson and Brianna Rapini, *The Amoeba Sisters' Cartoon Guide to Biology*. Mango Publishing Group, 2022.

INTERNET SOURCES

"Blood," *Nemours TeensHealth*, January 2019. https://kidshealth.org.

"Immune System Explained," *Better Health Channel*, July 18, 2022. www.betterhealth.vic.gov.au.

"Medical Laboratory Scientist," *Mayo Clinic*, n.d. https://college.mayo.edu.

WEBSITES

Science Journal for Kids and Teens

www.sciencejournalforkids.org

Science Journal for Kids and Teens contains articles about science topics in a variety of languages. Article topics include biology, health, chemistry, and more.

Science News Explores

www.snexplores.org

Science News Explores was founded in 2003. It publishes articles for young people about a wide range of science topics. The website has an entire section devoted to articles about health and medicine.

TeenLife

www.teenlife.com

TeenLife was created in 2007. Today, it provides teens with resources and tips to help them succeed in their future careers. The website contains information about different colleges, majors, and career paths.

INDEX

IMAGE CREDITS

Cover: © PeopleImages/Shutterstock Images
5: © NadyaTk/Shutterstock Images
7: © Fit Ztudio/Shutterstock Images
9: David Williams/Wikimedia Commons
10: © Wasan Tita/Shutterstock Images
13: © Ayo Production/Shutterstock Images
14: © Anakins srk/Shutterstock Images
17: © Dmytro Zinkevych/Shutterstock Images
19: © Svitlana Hulko/Shutterstock Images
20: © RHJPhtotos/Shutterstock Images
23: © Krakenimages.com/Shutterstock Images
24: © Komsan Loonprom/Shutterstock Images
27: © Katherine Welles/Shutterstock Images
29: © Koldo_Studio/Shutterstock Images
31: © Mangostar/Shutterstock Images
32: © S. Singha/Shutterstock Images
35: © Janthiwa Sutthiboriban/Shutterstock Images
36: © Creative Endeavors/Shutterstock Images
39: © Komsan Loonprom/Shutterstock Images
41: © CrizzyStudio/Shutterstock Images
42: © PeopleImages/Shutterstock Images
47: © fotovapl/Shutterstock Images
49: © PeopleImages/Shutterstock Images
50: © Gorodenkoff/Shutterstock Images
52: Red Line Editorial
55: © A Hip A Hub Stock/Shutterstock Images
56: © Hispanolistic/iStockphoto

ABOUT THE AUTHOR

Mike Downs is the author of more than thirty-five books for young people. He loves writing books that help people learn more about the world.